BEAT INSOMNIA QUICKLY

BULLET GUIDE

T0343118

Hodder Education, 338 Euston Road, London NW1 3BH

Hodder Education is an Hachette UK company

First published in UK 2012 by Hodder Education

This edition published 2012.

Copyright © 2012 Sara Kirkham

The moral rights of the author have been asserted.

Database right Hodder Education (makers)

Artworks (internal and cover): Peter Lubach

Cover concept design: Two Associates

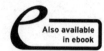

British Library Cataloguing in Publication Data: a catalogue record for this title is available from the British Library.

10 9 8 7 6 5 4 3 2 1

The publisher has used its best endeavours to ensure that any website addresses referred to in this book are correct and active at the time of going to press. However, the publisher and the author have no responsibility for the websites and can make no guarantee that a site will remain live or that the content will remain relevant, decent or appropriate.

The publisher has made every effort to mark as such all words which it believes to be trademarks. The publisher should also like to make it clear that the presence of a word in the book, whether marked or unmarked, in no way affects its legal status as a trademark.

Every reasonable effort has been made by the publisher to trace the copyright holders of material in this book. Any errors or omissions should be notified in writing to the publisher, who will endeavour to rectify the situation for any reprints and future editions.

Hachette UK's policy is to use papers that are natural, renewable and recyclable products and made from wood grown in sustainable forests. The logging and manufacturing processes are expected to conform to the environmental regulations of the country of origin.

www.hoddereducation.co.uk

Typeset by Stephen Rowling/Springworks

Printed in Spain

BEAT INSOMNIA QUICKLY

BULLET GUIDE

Sara Kirkham

About the author

Sara Kirkham is a nutritionist, writer and lecturer with over 20 years' experience of helping people to make lifestyle changes to improve their health. Sara has written many books and articles on health, lifestyle, diet and nutrition, and she has a First-class Honours degree in Nutritional Medicine.

As a nutritional therapist, Sara often sees clients with insomnia and uses a number of lifestyle adaptations including diet and exercise, as well as supplements and herbs, to help allay their insomnia or its underlying cause. Spending many years working alongside other complementary therapists, including those practising clinical hypnosis, has also given her a good working knowledge of how these therapies, as well as cognitive behavioural techniques, can help insomnia. With many years' experience of helping people to adapt their diet and lifestyle, Sara has captured all that practical information and expertise in *Beat Insomnia Quickly*, providing you with the most effective guide to getting a good night's sleep.

Contents

1 All about insomnia   1
2 All about sleep   13
3 Lifestyle causes of insomnia   25
4 How your health affects your sleep   37
5 What can I take for insomnia?   49
6 Is your diet keeping you awake?   61
7 Learning to 'switch off'   73
8 Alternative therapies   85
9 Herbs to help   97
10 Perfect sleep plan   109

Introduction

Almost everyone has problems sleeping at some point, with up to 50% of us experiencing bouts of insomnia and 10% suffering with chronic insomnia. Whether your insomnia is temporary, caused by passing events such as exams or recovery from an operation, in response to something specific such as the menopause or pregnancy, or chronic with no known cause, *Beat Insomnia Quickly* will help you to explore potential reasons for your disrupted sleep and show you how to remedy it.

Beat Insomnia Quickly provides you with a succinct and easy to understand guide to what causes insomnia. It explores the treatment options, including a wealth of practical tips, giving you all the tools you need to conquer your insomnia.

In this guide you will discover:

* information on different types of insomnia
* the most common causes of insomnia

* what sleep is, why we need it and how much you need
* ways to help you identify what may be causing your insomnia
* help to improve insomnia during pregnancy and the menopause
* ways to tackle insomnia caused by medical conditions, such as restless legs syndrome or sleep apnoea
* practical tips to improve insomnia caused by lifestyle habits
* what to eat – and what foods to avoid – to get a good night's sleep
* suggestions to help insomnia caused by psychological factors (e.g. stress)
* unbiased information on over-the-counter and prescription sleeping medication
* alternative treatment options for insomnia
* tips on which herbs to try and how to use them
* the ultimate perfect sleep plan – including what to do during the day, pre-bedtime rituals that encourage sleep and tips to get you back to sleep if you do wake up during the night.

Beat Insomnia Quickly – guaranteed to give you a good night's sleep!

1 All about insomnia

Insomnia is **difficulty in getting to sleep and/or staying asleep**. It can also mean feeling as if you **haven't slept well**. Almost everyone has problems sleeping at some point, with up to 50% of us experiencing bouts of insomnia and 10% suffering from chronic insomnia.

As we all differ in our need for sleep, insomnia is recognized as a **disruption to a normal sleep pattern**, rather than being defined as lacking a specific number of hours of sleep.

You are more likely to experience insomnia if you are:

* adolescent
* female
* pregnant or menopausal.

Insomnia can be either a lack of *quality* sleep or a lack of *quantity* of sleep

Types of insomnia

* Sleep-onset insomnia (can't get to sleep)
* Waking during the night
* Not feeling refreshed after sleep
* Waking up too early

Naturally, a lack of sleep affects how well you function throughout the day, and can cause sleepiness and irritability.

Inability to sleep well is often transient, or **short-term, insomnia**, but if you have trouble sleeping for more than 3 weeks, this is known as **chronic insomnia**.

The most important thing is to try to discover the cause of your inability to get a good night's sleep.

In this chapter you will learn more about the various types and causes of insomnia.

Causes of insomnia

There are many possible causes of insomnia, and the cause is often linked to the duration. For example, **lifestyle or situational factors** cause short-term insomnia only for as long as they exist:

* noise
* light
* room temperature
* caffeine, nicotine, alcohol or drugs
* change in sleeping location (new house, holiday)
* jet lag

* changes in shift work
* physical conditions such as nasal congestion
* medication
* stressful events
* withdrawal from a drug.

In these cases, dealing with the cause of your insomnia should improve your sleep pattern.

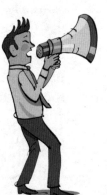

● Loud or irritating noises can prevent you getting a good night's sleep

4

Although emotional problems or difficulties at work may cause stress and sleeplessness only while the issue lasts, this may be long enough to affect your sleep pattern and overall health. Underlying **psychological, psychiatric** or **medical conditions** are often linked with chronic insomnia.

Psychological causes of insomnia

* Worry
* Anxiety
* Depression
* Stress (mental, emotional, situational)
* Schizophrenia
* Bipolar disorder

People with anxiety or depression are significantly more likely to develop insomnia

Physiological causes of insomnia

Physical conditions – and/or the medication taken for them – can cause short- or long-term insomnia. Common conditions include:

* chronic pain
* chronic fatigue syndrome (ME)
* acid reflux
* nocturnal hypoglycaemia (low blood sugar)
* sleep apnoea
* joint or muscle problems such as arthritis, fibromyalgia or restless legs syndrome

* incontinence or enlarged prostate gland
* neurotransmitter imbalance
* hormone imbalance (such as during pregnancy or menopause)
* night-time breathing problems.

Insomnia may also be a symptom or result of respiratory disease, angina or stroke, an overactive thyroid gland, Parkinson's or Alzheimer's disease or a brain tumour.

Insomnia is not a disease, but a symptom or result of some other condition or cause

Insomnia during pregnancy

Insomnia can also occur at certain times of life, most notably during **pregnancy** and the **menopause**.

Pregnancy generally increases sleep requirements but insomnia during pregnancy affects up to 80% of women. Here are some common causes and suggested solutions.

Can't get comfortable in bed?

Inability to get **comfortable** or **back strain** due to a 'bump' at the front altering your centre of balance can cause sleepless nights. Reduce backache by:

- ☑ wearing flat or low-heeled shoes during the day
- ☑ sleeping on your left side and putting pillows under your bump, between your legs and under your lower back
- ☑ having a massage to ease muscle tension.

Waking up because of dreams, stress or anxiety

Increased levels of **oestrogen** and **progesterone** during pregnancy can increase the amount of rapid eye movement (REM) sleep, so you **dream** more. Try to alleviate stress and anxiety in the evenings before bedtime and you will reduce the chance of having vivid or nightmarish dreams.

Although homeopathic or herbal remedies may be used during pregnancy with the guidance of a qualified practitioner, you may wish to try gentler **Bach or other flower remedies**. These are very dilute preparations of botanical essences, which some people find comforting:

* To reduce stress and tension try **Bach Rescue Remedy**.
* If vivid dreams are waking you, try **Bach Mimulus** or **Rock Rose**.

8

Restless legs syndrome

Even if you have not been diagnosed with **pregnancy anaemia** (low iron levels), you may still require additional iron to prevent restless legs syndrome. Iron requirements during pregnancy increase, so try taking a pregnancy multivitamin/-mineral and eating plenty of **green leafy vegetables, lean meats, lentils** and **dried apricots**. This condition has also been linked with an increased requirement for **folic acid**, the daily requirement for which doubles from 200 to 400 micrograms during pregnancy. As well as ensuring that you get this amount with a supplement, make sure that you include foods rich in folic acid in your diet, for example **raspberries, brown rice, granary bread** and **green leafy vegetables**.

Other problems associated with pregnancy

Leg cramps may be caused in the later stages of pregnancy by the additional weight straining your leg muscles. Try stretching out the calf muscles before bed by sitting with your legs straight out in front of you, bringing the toes up towards your shins and pressing your heels away from you, and holding this for 20–30 seconds.

To reduce **heartburn** try raising the head end of the bed on bricks, and avoid eating late, large amounts or spicy foods.

A growing foetus can put pressure on the **bladder**, causing more frequent urination. Stay well hydrated throughout the day but **reduce fluid intake in the evening** to reduce the likelihood of having to wake up to visit the bathroom.

10

Insomnia during the menopause

Insomnia during the **menopause** can be caused by declining hormone levels with resultant **hot flushes** and **night sweats**. If your insomnia is hormone related but you don't want to take **hormone replacement therapy** (HRT), try:

* Keeping your bedroom **cooler** to reduce **night sweats**.
* Eating lots of natural **phyto- (plant) oestrogens** to rebalance hormone levels, such as soya products, apples, plums, cherries, peppers, yams, tomatoes, olives, carrots, fennel, potatoes and aubergine.
* Filling up on foods rich in **vitamin E**: nuts, seeds, avocado, wheatgerm and pine nuts.
* Taking **isoflavone supplements** to boost natural oestrogen levels.
* Taking a **multivitamin/-mineral supplement** to rebalance nutrient levels, especially those minerals affected by the menopause such as magnesium and calcium.

2 All about sleep

Sleep is a state of consciousness that allows us to rest and rejuvenate. Sleep is largely regulated by **neurotransmitters** (chemicals in the nervous system) which control our **sleep/wake cycle** in response to exposure to **light** or **darkness**.

Serotonin (a neurotransmitter) is converted into **melatonin**, which is secreted into the bloodstream at night and creates **drowsiness**. Melatonin levels usually stay high for 12 hours, but upon exposure to artificial light or sunlight, melatonin secretion drops and we wake up.

The body clock is a biological cycle called the circadian rhythm – this controls waking and sleeping

Many bodily functions, including body temperature and our sleep pattern, follow the biological cycle known as the **circadian cycle or rhythm**. Jet lag is the feeling we get when this cycle has been disrupted; shift workers may experience similar feelings as their lifestyle conflicts with natural cues such as sunlight and normal meal times.

Although we might use an alarm clock to set our **waking time**, light and body temperature naturally control our sleep rhythm. Temperature peaks and troughs are thought to mirror our sleep pattern: **body temperature** is higher during daytime and lower at night when we drop off to sleep.

In this chapter you will learn more about the sleep cycle and the different stages of sleep.

Why do we need sleep?

In order to function properly and remain healthy, we need **regular sleep**. Anyone who has experienced insomnia knows how debilitating lack of sleep can be. Just look at the most likely symptoms of missing a night's sleep:

* drowsiness
* inability to focus
* poor concentration
* irritability
* impaired memory
* slower reaction time
* impaired physical performance.

Sleep deprivation also results in **depressed immune function**, making us more susceptible to infection and illness, and we may feel cold as **body temperature drops** when we are tired.

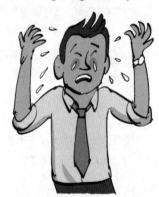

● Lack of sleep affects our emotional state

How much sleep do we need?

Far from being a passive state, the brain and body are very active during sleep. Sleep is when our body forms essential hormones and antibodies, repairs body cells and promotes growth. Parts of the brain that control emotions and social interaction are rested, enabling us to function better when we are awake.

We all need different amounts of sleep – this is affected by age and lifestyle and also changes throughout life. The amount of sleep needed also depends on whether we have been deprived of sleep in previous days, creating a **sleep debt**. This is commonly called '**catching up on sleep**'.

Sleep through the ages

We need **different amounts of sleep** at different times in our life.
During growth phases from babyhood through childhood to puberty, we
require more sleep to enable our body to grow.

Newborn babies may sleep for 18 hours a day.

Toddlers sleep for 14–18 hours daily.

Growing children need 11–13 hours' sleep.

Average adults sleep for 7–9 hours a night.

Older people, over 70, usually need less than 6 hours' sleep.

For most adults, sleep **of 8–8.4 hours** is considered **fully restorative**, although an individual may require anything between 5 and 10 hours daily. Some cultures divide total sleep time into a **siesta** of 1–2 hours and an overnight sleep of 6–7 hours.

We tend to **sleep less** and **more lightly** as we age – time spent in light sleep may increase by 5% compared with young adults, but deep sleep decreases by 10–15%, reducing overall sleep time. It can also take older adults longer to fall to sleep, so it's a good idea to make up for lost sleep with **daytime naps** as we get older.

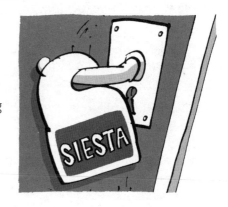

Sleep stages and the sleep cycle

During sleep the body goes through different **sleep stages** in a cycle lasting approximately 90 minutes. After **drowsiness**, the **sleep stages** can be described as:

* light sleep (stage 1)
* stage 2 (moving from light to deep sleep)
* deep sleep (stages 3 and 4)
* dreaming (REM sleep).

After the REM phase, we begin the cycle again, going through **five cycles** in a night.

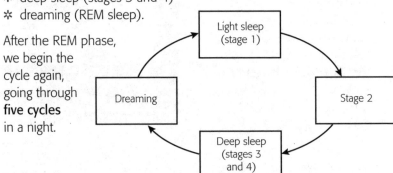

A normal night's sleep can be divided into three equal time periods, as we generally spend more time in **lighter stages of sleep** in the earlier part of the night, and more time in **deep sleep** and **REM sleep** later on:

Types of sleep

1 Sleep in the first third of the night comprises mostly non-REM sleep (stages 1 to 4).
2 Sleep in the middle third of the night includes a little more REM sleep.
3 Sleep in the last third of the night is mostly REM sleep.

We normally awake from a full night's sleep from REM sleep.

Sleep is a complicated physiological phenomenon that scientists do not fully understand

Non-REM sleep (stages 1–4)

Stage 1 (light sleep) is the transition between being awake and asleep. This stage occurs when we initially fall asleep and in arousal periods during sleep, accounting for 5–10% of total sleep time. We can be easily awakened during this stage.

Stage 2 is 40–50% of total sleep time. Brain waves slow down with occasional bursts of nerve activity. Eye movement stops during this stage.

In **stage 3** slow brain waves are interspersed with smaller, faster waves. In **stage 4** slow brain waves predominate. Stages 3 and 4 together represent approximately 20% of total sleep time and are called **deep sleep**. Eye and muscle movement stops and it is difficult to wake someone during these stages.

Sleep.walking, bedwetting and nightmares are usually experienced during deep sleep.

REM sleep

This represents 20–25% of total sleep time, occurring four to five times during a typical 8-hour sleep. The first REM period of the night may last less than 10 minutes, the last may exceed 60 minutes. In a normal night's sleep, bouts of REM sleep occur every 90 minutes, but if we are very sleepy, the duration of REM sleep may be very short or it may even be absent.

REM sleep is usually associated with **dreaming**. The brain is highly active with similar brain wave activity to wakefulness, but during REM sleep:

* The eyeballs move rapidly.
* The heart rate and breathing become rapid and irregular.
* The blood pressure rises.
* The muscles are virtually paralysed.

3 Lifestyle causes of insomnia

Most of us experience trouble sleeping at some point, and whether or not this turns into chronic insomnia will depend upon whether the cause is **transient** and whether you identify the **cause** and do something about it.

Insomnia may be caused by things that you can change:

* room temperature
* noise
* mattress and/or bed clothes
* light
* jet lag
* changes in shift work
* caffeine, nicotine, alcohol or drugs
* change in sleeping location (new house, holiday)
* physical conditions such as nasal congestion
* medication
* stress or overactive mind
* withdrawal from a drug.

In this chapter you will learn about the things that can affect your sleep and how to change them.

Room temperature

The bedroom temperature should be **18–24°C** and feel **cool**. If it is too hot or too cold, this can easily prevent or disrupt sleep. Check this list:

Too hot	Too cold
Reduce bedding layers	Increase bedding layers
Use lighter cotton sheets/thinner duvet	Use thicker duvet
Open windows – if too noisy, ventilate through the day to cool the room	Turn up heating
Sleep in the buff!	Close windows and doors
Sleep in a bigger, better ventilated room	Sleep in a warmer room
Switch off/turn down heating	Heat house through before bedtime
Sleep alone to reduce body heat	Wear thicker nightclothes, bed socks, a hat
Get a fan	Snuggle up to your partner for warmth

Noise

Noise can stop you from getting to sleep and may wake you during the night or early in the morning. Common noise pollutants include:

* noise from snoring bed partner or other family members
* noisy neighbours' voices, music, cars, doors slamming
* traffic noise (road, air or rail)
* industrial noise from generators, roadworks, etc.
* pets – yours or other people's
* birds.

Being kept awake or woken up by any of these is initially irritating, but, if it happens on a daily basis, it can lead to chronic insomnia. So what can you do about it?

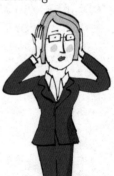

● Noise is a common cause of insomnia

Strategies for silencing noise

Animals and birds
Double glazing
Birds in loft/on roof, call RSPB
Ear plugs
Sleep in another room

Traffic and industrial noise
Double glazing
Ear plugs
Sleep in another room
Listen to low-level music/relaxation CD to drown out other noise but induce sleep

Noise

In the house – TV, music, etc.
Turn TV/music volume down
Close all doors
Can listener wear headphones?
Move noise further away
Sound proofing – heavy curtains over doorways
Ear plugs
Sleep in another room
Agree a music/TV time curfew

Noise outside
Close windows
Double glazing
Speak to neighbours/notify the council
Ear plugs
Sleep in another room
Listen to low-level music/relaxation CD to drown out other noise but induce sleep

Check your mattress

If your **mattress** is too old, too soft or too hard it may be affecting your sleep. We shed approximately **500 grams of skin** yearly (much of it in bed) and almost **300 millilitres of sweat** nightly, so bedding and mattresses need regular cleaning. Bedding can also contribute to allergies such as asthma, so it's worth a **spring clean**:

* Turn your mattress over and around for even wear.
* Strip the bed regularly, and open the windows to ventilate the mattress.
* Dust the bed base and around the bed.
* Wash pillows, duvets and blankets.
* Fit a washable, hypoallergenic mattress cover to keep the mattress clean and deter dust mites.
* Consider whether you need an orthopaedic or 'memory' mattress.

A good-quality mattress and bed frame will give you an extra hour's sleep each night.

The Sleep Council

Light

It is natural to wake with the **sunlight**, but this may not suit your schedule, and, during summer in an **east-facing** room with thin curtains, you may be woken daily at 4 am!

Other sources of unwanted light include **street lights** or **security lights**.

So how can you trick your **body clock** into thinking it's not yet time to get up?

- ☑ Get thicker curtains or blackout blinds.
- ☑ Wear an eye mask.
- ☑ If a security light is shining into your bedroom, could it be diverted away?
- ☑ Change the position of your bed so that you are not facing the window.

Resetting the body clock

Sleep is largely regulated by **light/darkness** picked up through the eyes: when exposed to light, melatonin levels drop and we begin to wake up, regardless of the time. **Shift work** or **long-haul flights** affect our natural **body clock**, as we are trying to sleep and wake at times different from our usual routine, which can cause insomnia.

☑ Use bright light and darkness to reset your body clock.
☑ Make use of ear plugs and eye masks if trying to sleep during the day.
☑ Stick to the same wake and sleep times on days off work, rather than adjusting your body clock again.

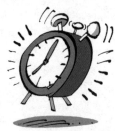

32

Switching off

An 'overactive mind', worrying or stress are common factors that may prevent sleep. **Winding down** before bedtime and having a **pre-sleep ritual** can help you to sleep. Create your own bedtime ritual from these tips to help you 'drop off':

* Go to bed at the same time each night.
* Avoid stimulants such as caffeine, nicotine and alcohol.
* Take a warm (not hot) bath.
* Relax the muscles with gentle stretching.
* Listen to relaxation CDs, audiobooks or relaxing sound effects.
* Write a 'to do' list for the next day to help clear your mind.
* Distract yourself by reading or listening to music or the radio.
* Have some sort of 'white noise' in the background, such as a room fan.

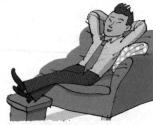

● Relax at the end of the evening in a dim room

Creating a relaxing environment for sleep

Just as a busy mind can prevent sleep, so can a 'busy' or untidy room. As well as being **cool, quiet** and **dark**, your bedroom should be **tidy** and not used for other activities such as watching TV. Even using a mobile phone before bedtime may interfere with sleep patterns, according to a study by Professor Arnetz at the Karolinska Institute, Stockholm, and colleagues at Wayne State University, Detroit, published in 2007.

Studies have shown that **colours** may affect our mood, so consider your bedroom décor and choose a restful colour to help you get a good night's sleep.

* **Purple** is calming for the mind and body.
* **Green** can create peace and serenity, reducing stress.
* **Blue** encourages daydreaming, and prompts the release of sleep hormones.
* **Neutral** colours may help us to wind down.

Lifestyle check

Several lifestyle habits may help or hinder sleep.

Exercise

Regular exercise promotes physical tiredness and better sleep. However, vigorous exercise stimulates the sympathetic nervous system, and so shouldn't be done too late in the evening (or too close to sleep).

Sex

Hormones such as **oxytocin,** produced during sex, induce feelings of well-being and drowsiness, and can help promote a good night's sleep.

Smoking

Nicotine is a stimulant, and smokers often sleep very lightly, missing restorative REM sleep. Heavy smokers may even be woken by nicotine withdrawal symptoms after a few hours.

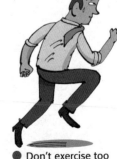

● Don't exercise too late in the day

4 How your health affects your sleep

Just as lack of sleep affects our health, our health can affect our sleep. If a health condition is affecting your sleep, target the **physical cause** of your insomnia, rather than reach for the sleeping pills. You may find a simple remedy to your problem, or you may need to see your doctor or a sleep specialist.

Physical causes include:

* chronic pain
* joint or muscle problems
* restless legs syndrome
* acid reflux
* nocturnal hypoglycaemia (low blood sugar)
* sleep apnoea.

Restless legs syndrome is a cause of sleep impairment in 5–10% of the population in the USA

In this chapter, you will learn about the ways in which your health can affect your sleep.

Pain

Using **painkillers** for temporary conditions may enable you to sleep, but it is better to treat the cause of the problem rather than the symptom.

If you can pinpoint the cause of your insomnia, find tips in this book to help:

* For stress, try relaxation or meditation techniques.
* Try a more supportive or memory mattress.
* Natural anti-inflammatories and analgesics, prescribed by a qualified nutritional therapist or herbalist, may reduce pain without drug side effects.

Restless legs syndrome

This is the fourth most common cause of insomnia, and severe cases result in the greatest sleep deprivation of any sleep disorder. It is characterized by a compulsion to keep moving the legs at night. It can be caused by **impaired dopamine metabolism** (dopamine is a neurotransmitter) or **iron deficiency**, and may respond to additional **folic acid**, **magnesium** or **vitamin E** in the diet.

Foods rich in:			
Iron	Magnesium	Folic acid	Vitamin E
Meat	Cauliflower	Raspberries	Nuts
Seafood	Banana	Salmon	Seeds
Eggs	Nuts	Leafy veg	Avocado
Leafy veg	Pulses	Beans	Wheat germ

For a **sleep-inducing supper**, try porridge with milk and added raspberries, pumpkin seeds and flaked almonds.

Restless legs syndrome may also respond to several other dietary and lifestyle adjustments:

- ☑ limit refined carbohydrates and sugary foods
- ☑ reduce caffeine intake
- ☑ stop smoking
- ☑ reduce alcohol intake.

Medications that may induce or worsen restless legs syndrome include several prescribed for depression:

- ✳ selective serotonin re-uptake inhibitors (SSRIs)
- ✳ lithium
- ✳ dopamine agonists
- ✳ tricyclic antidepressants
- ✳ antiemetics
- ✳ antipsychotics.

Blood iron concentrations have a circadian rhythm, falling by up to 60% at night compared with daytime levels, and these drops are correlated with the severity of restless legs syndrome

Acid reflux

If **acid reflux** keeps you awake at night, before you reach for the indigestion remedy or sleeping pills, try these tips, which may reduce indigestion and solve the problem:

1 Avoid eating late at night.
2 Avoid large meals.
3 Chew food thoroughly.
4 Make the evening meal low fat (no cream, cheese or creamy puddings).
5 Keep protein intake low (limit meat, fish, eggs, soya and dairy products).
6 Avoid spicy foods.
7 Avoid alcohol, tea and coffee.
8 Try excluding foods you may be intolerant to, such as wheat, dairy or eggs.

TOP TIP
Raising the head end of the bed on bricks can help to stop acid reflux at night.

Try a mug of **chamomile tea** at night – it may help to ease heartburn and also has sedative properties to help you sleep.

Nocturnal hypoglycaemia

If you are waking up during the night hungry, you may have **nocturnal hypoglycaemia** (night-time low blood sugar). It may be up to 12 hours between dinner and 'breaking the fast' at breakfast, and if **blood sugar levels** drop too low while you are asleep, this can wake you up. Tips to help:

☑ Have **slow-release carbohydrates**, such as brown rice, wholemeal pasta or pulses, in your evening meal.

☑ Have an **oat-based sleep-inducing supper**, such as an oat cereal bar with a glass of milk or a bowl of milky porridge with tryptophan-rich bananas and almonds containing calcium and magnesium.

☑ **Avoid sugary or refined carbohydrates** or caffeinated products, as the initial peak in blood sugar may be followed by hypoglycaemia as insulin is released to reduce blood sugar levels.

Sleep apnoea

Snoring, as well as contributing to a partner's sleepless nights, can also be a sign of **sleep apnoea**, a sleeping disorder in which the breathing repeatedly stops and starts. It often goes unrecognized, but left untreated can be detrimental to health, causing diabetes, hypertension, heart disease and weight gain. In sleep apnoea, phases of breathing are **shallow** or **interrupted** throughout the night. **Blood oxygen levels** drop and so the brain disturbs your sleep to kick-start breathing. You may not remember these brief 'awakenings', but it stops you from getting a good night's sleep – your natural sleep rhythm is disturbed and you spend more time in light sleep and less time in deep, restorative sleep. This leaves you with daytime sleepiness, slow reflexes and poor concentration.

You may need to stay at a sleep clinic for sleep apnoea to be diagnosed

Snorting or snoring may wake you up during the night, but, if it doesn't, you (or your partner) might recognize these other symptoms of sleep apnoea:

* gasping or breathing pauses
* going to the bathroom frequently
* daytime sleepiness, irritability or difficulty in concentrating
* waking up with a dry mouth, sore throat or headache, or feeling out of breath.

There are different types of sleep apnoea:

* **Obstructive sleep apnoea** Soft tissue at the back of the throat relaxes during sleep and blocks the airway, causing snoring.
* **Central sleep apnoea** The brain fails to control the breathing muscles.
* **Complex sleep apnoea** A combination of obstructive and central sleep apnoea.

Causes of sleep apnoea

Central sleep apnoea is often linked with illness, but risk factors for **obstructive sleep apnoea** include:

* being overweight
* smoking
* male
* aged over 65
* black, Hispanic, or a Pacific Islander
* a family history of sleep apnoea
* allergies causing nasal congestion.

You can't change your gender, race or age, but **stopping smoking** and **losing weight** will reduce your risk of sleep apnoea, as will identifying **allergies** and taking steps to remedy them. Avoid sedatives, sleeping pills and alcohol as they relax the throat muscles and may exacerbate sleep apnoea.

46

Tips for preventing sleep apnoea

* **Sleep on your side** – your tongue is less likely to obstruct your airway.
* **Prop your head up**, sleep on a **foam wedge** or elevate the top half of the bed if you can.
* Open nasal passages at night by wearing a **breathing strip** or using a **saline spray**.
* Sew a **tennis ball** into the back of your pyjamas or into a pillow behind your back to stop you rolling on to your back during the night.

TOP TIP
Breathing strips, cervical pillows, foam wedges and continuous positive airflow pressure devices are all available from sleep specialists, or on prescription, to help reduce sleep apnoea.

5 What can I take for insomnia?

The idea of a pill that promises a **good night's sleep** is very appealing, but taking sleeping pills treats the symptom (the insomnia) and not the **cause**. Although over-the-counter and prescription sleep medications may help you to sleep, they don't cure the underlying cause, and may even worsen insomnia. Considerations of taking sleeping pills include:

* side effects
* drug tolerance
* drug dependence
* withdrawal symptoms
* interactions with other drugs, herbs or supplements
* masking an underlying problem.

Rebound insomnia is when you stop taking sleeping drugs and the insomnia returns worse than before

You may find that you have to increase the dosage of sleeping medication for it to remain effective, leading to side effects and increasing the risk of dependency. Any type of sleeping medication is more effective when used **as and when required**, rather than every day when it will begin to become less effective as the body becomes accustomed to it, following which **dependency** and **addiction** may occur. These medications are best used for **short-term situations**, such as to prevent jet lag or during recovery from an operation. There are many remedies available **over the counter**, but these are sometimes ineffective and, if dosages higher than those recommended are taken, they can be dangerous.

In this chapter you will learn about the medications available for insomnia and also how other medications can contribute to insomnia.

Over-the-counter medications

5-Hydroxytryptophan (5-HTP)

Medical research indicates that taking 1 gram of **L-tryptophan** before bedtime can induce sleepiness and delay waking time. Researchers believe that L-tryptophan initiates sleep by raising **serotonin** levels, a chemical that promotes relaxation. However, tryptophan can interact adversely with certain antidepressants and cause serious negative side effects, so **5-hydroxytryptophan (5-HTP)** is a safer option.

Studies suggest that 5-HTP, made from tryptophan (an amino acid found in protein-rich foods) may be useful in treating insomnia associated with **depression**. Interactions with drugs – particularly antidepressants – can occur, so always consult a health professional before taking 5-HTP supplements.

52

Melatonin

Melatonin is a hormone that plays a critical role in our **sleep/wake cycle** and other **circadian rhythms**. Research conducted at the University of Alberta examined 17 studies with 651 people and found no significant side effects when melatonin was used for 3 months or less, but long-term effects and the efficacy of melatonin supplementation are not known, and further testing is required to ascertain its safety. Experts **caution** that you should not take melatonin supplements if you have depression, schizophrenia, an autoimmune disease or other serious illness, or are pregnant or breastfeeding.

TOP TIP
Some research has shown that you may boost your melatonin levels naturally by meditating before bedtime.

Antihistamines

Antihistamines such as Benadryl, Dreemon, Night-calm, NyQuil or Nytol may be used for short-term insomnia, but **side effects** can include a dry mouth, hangover-type symptoms and sedative effects during the day. These medications may help to promote sleep in the short term but are not recommended for insomnia lasting more than 4 weeks. Long-term use may cause **addiction**, and is not dealing with the cause of the insomnia.

54

Tips for using over-the-counter sleeping drugs

Check for any contraindications for use – for example, don't use during pregnancy or while breast feeding.

Start with the smallest dose.

Take medication about half an hour before bedtime (or as instructed).

Prescription medications

Side effects

Taking prescription medications may be your best option if you know what the cause of your insomnia is, but cannot change or treat it. In this way, at least you will be getting more sleep. However, sleeping pills can cause side effects such as:

* drowsiness and fatigue during the day
* dizziness and nausea
* blurred vision
* clumsiness and problems with balance
* dry mouth and throat
* impaired concentration and co-ordination
* confusion and disorientation
* memory problems
* anxiety and depression
* irritability
* panic attacks, paranoia or hallucinations
* irregular heart beat.

Pros and cons

Prescription medications for insomnia may be more effective than over-the-counter remedies, but can also cause **dependence**, and coming off the drug involves slowly reducing the dosage to avoid withdrawal symptoms.

Sleeping medications generally act by affecting receptors in the brain to **slow down** the nervous system. Some drugs induce sleep; others maintain sleep.

Older medications may have more research behind them, but newer ones may have fewer side effects and a better safety profile, so, if you have been taking the same sleeping medication for a while, it may be worth checking with your doctor to see if there is a better option for you.

56

Types of prescription sleeping medication

Before prescribing sleeping tablets, your doctor may refer you to a **clinical psychologist** or **sleep specialist** to try to determine the cause of your insomnia. If various non-drug interventions such as **cognitive behavioural therapy** fail to help, your doctor may prescribe sleeping pills:

* if your symptoms are particularly severe
* to ease short-term insomnia.

Benzodiazepines

These are tranquillizers designed to reduce anxiety, and are the oldest class of sleep medications still commonly prescribed. These drugs are thought to have a higher risk of dependence than other sedative hypnotics used to treat insomnia. Drawbacks include dependency, withdrawal symptoms, rebound insomnia, poor sleep quality and daytime drowsiness.

Z medicines (non-benzodiazepines)

These work in a similar way to benzodiazepines, but are a newer type of drug thought to have fewer side effects and less risk of dependency. However, side effects still include daytime drowsiness and the risk of tolerance, dependency and withdrawal symptoms.

Melatonin agonists

These promote the onset of sleep by increasing levels of melatonin, which helps to normalize the **circadian rhythm** and sleep/wake cycle. There appear to be fewer side effects with this type of medication, and little risk of dependency. However, this type of drug is more effective for the treatment of sleep-onset problems rather than helping to keep you asleep.

58

Insomnia as a drug side effect

Insomnia is one of the most common **side effects** of taking other medications. Medicines known to cause insomnia include:

* steroids
* non-steroidal anti-inflammatories
* beta blockers
* thyroid hormones
* nasal decongestants
* appetite suppressants/diet pills containing caffeine
* asthma medication
* epilepsy medication
* hormone treatment
* antidepressants
* stimulant drugs used to treat conditions such as attention deficit disorder.

It is essential that you do not stop taking medication without consulting your doctor, but if you suffer from insomnia, check with your doctor to see if your medication could be causing it and whether there are any suitable alternatives. After all, lack of sleep is not going to help your health!

6 Is your diet keeping you awake?

Perhaps because insomnia is known to be a symptom of something and not an illness in its own right, most people try **self-care** or **natural or traditional remedies** before going to see their doctor. There is much folklore and many 'traditional' remedies for a good night's sleep, but do they work?

Having a **warm milky drink** is a well-known remedy to aid sleep, but although the milk contains **tryptophan** (which converts into serotonin, which in turn is converted into melatonin, which helps us sleep), and minerals calcium and magnesium (also linked with better sleep), many people don't find this helpful for insomnia.

Historically, nutmeg was used as a sleep remedy in India and Malaysia

In this chapter, you will learn how to change your diet to give you the best chance of a good night's sleep.

Another folk remedy is to add a little **nutmeg** to a milky drink. Nutmeg contains a chemical that reduces the breakdown of **serotonin** – a neurotransmitter converted into melatonin to induce sleep – so there may be some substance to this traditional remedy.

However, '**night caps**' such as whisky may not help – alcohol is a sedative, but has a rebound effect later on – it may help you get to sleep, but affects sleep detrimentally later on.

TOP TIP
Try mashed banana with ¼ teaspoon of freshly grated nutmeg and warm milk – the combination of sleep-inducing nutrients and nutmeg's magical ingredient may just do the job!

Foods that can contribute to insomnia

We often forget about the **stimulant** effect of many foods and drinks, which can keep us awake at night. Most people know that caffeine is a stimulant, yet we often fail to think about how changing our daily habits could effectively prevent insomnia. Your sleeplessness could be the result of something as simple as too much **caffeine**, too late in the day.

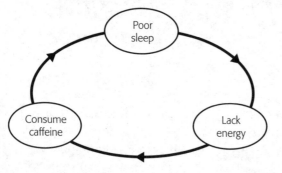

Poor sleep → Lack energy → Consume caffeine →

Save the (caffeine-filled) chocolate on your pillow for a daytime snack.
National Sleep Foundation

The main foods that can contribute to insomnia are:

* caffeine-containing drinks – coffee, tea, hot chocolate and energy drinks
* chocolate
* sugary foods
* spicy foods.

In addition, **eating too late** can have an adverse effect upon sleep, causing indigestion or acid reflux if you lie down to sleep too soon after eating. Not eating enough can also wake you in the night – this drop in **blood sugar**, which will wake you up to snack on sugary drinks or food, is called **nocturnal hypoglycaemia** – and eating foods that don't agree with you can keep you awake with **indigestion**. The trick is to eat the right types of foods at the right time of day.

Caffeine

Making sure that **caffeine** is not to blame for your insomnia should be one of your first objectives. Caffeine is a stimulant, which can be useful during the day, but the **half-life of caffeine** in your body is approximately 6 hours, so, if you consume 100 mg of caffeine at 4 pm, you will still have 50 mg in your body at 10 pm.

Drink/food	Caffeine content
Instant coffee	50–100 mg per cup
Filter coffee	60–120 mg per cup
Tea	30–60 mg per cup
Green tea	10–20 mg per cup
Cola	Approximately 45 mg per can
Chocolate	80 mg per 100 g bar

You may benefit from keeping a **food/drink diary**, noting the times and amounts of caffeinated drinks you consume throughout the day in conjunction with your sleep pattern. If there is a link between caffeine intake and poor sleep, it's time to switch to decaffeinated drinks – although these can still contain 3–10 mg of caffeine.

Try these tips to reduce caffeine intake:

* Switch to decaffeinated coffee.
* Avoid caffeine after lunchtime.
* Drink weaker cups of coffee/tea.
* Drink tea instead of coffee.
* Drink green, rooibos (redbush) or herbal teas.
* Try herbal teas that promote sleep, such as chamomile.
* Don't eat chocolate or chocolatey foods at night.

A small bar of dark chocolate can contain more caffeine than a cup of instant coffee, so imagine the combined effects of coffee and chocolate!

Alcohol

Alcohol has a **sedative effect** so may seem to make you drowsy, but it deprives you of deep, restorative sleep, leaving you tired the next day. Heavy alcohol consumption can contribute to chronic insomnia by affecting your sleep pattern – you spend longer in **light sleep** and are more likely to wake up. Also, alcohol-induced thirst, needing to visit the bathroom or headaches can wake you up during the night.

To reduce alcohol intake:

- ☑ Alternate alcoholic drinks with a glass of water or juice.
- ☑ Add soda or extra mixers to alcohol to make the drink last longer.
- ☑ Make sure that you are well hydrated before you start drinking.
- ☑ Have alcohol-free days.
- ☑ Count how many units/alcoholic drinks you have each week, then set yourself a lower limit – and stick to it! The NHS recommends drinking no more than 2–3 units daily (women) or 3–4 units daily (men).

Correcting imbalances

Iron, folate, magnesium and vitamin E

A balanced diet is essential for healthy sleep. Deficiencies in or increased requirements for **iron** and **folate** are linked with **restless legs syndrome**, and sufferers may also benefit from additional **magnesium** and **vitamin E**. Research has found that insomniacs suffering from restless legs syndrome who increased their intake of these nutrients saw improvements in their sleep.

1 Make sure that you eat a **healthy balanced diet** containing eggs, beans, pulses, whole grains, dark-green leafy vegetables, wheat bran, nuts, brown rice and fruit to ensure adequate intake of these nutrients.
2 Try taking a **multivitamin/-mineral supplement** to fill any nutrient gaps in your diet.
3 If you still can't sleep, consult a qualified nutritional therapist who will ensure that your diet is balanced, suggest reducing stimulants and provide supplement advice.

Zinc and copper

One cause of insomnia specifically linked to diet is an unbalanced ratio between the minerals **zinc** and **copper**. Too much copper and/or too little zinc in the diet over a prolonged period can cause **heightened brain activity,** which keeps us awake, although zinc deficiency is more likely than too much copper. Certain factors increase the likelihood of zinc deficiency – if these apply to you, you may benefit from more zinc in your diet:

* long-term use of the contraceptive pill
* smoking
* alcohol consumption
* chronic stress
* a vegetarian diet.

Zinc-rich foods
Oysters, whole grains, pumpkin seeds, meat and offal

Tryptophan

Some nutrients in food promote a good night's sleep. Sleep is induced by **neurotransmitters** in the brain. **Serotonin** is a neurotransmitter formed from **tryptophan**, and serotonin forms **melatonin**, the neurotransmitter that initiates sleep. Therefore, eating tryptophan-rich foods can increase serotonin – and therefore **melatonin** – concentrations in the brain.

Tryptophan-rich foods

* Turkey
* Chicken
* Avocados
* Bananas
* Broccoli
* Spinach

For supper, combine **slow-release carbohydrates** and **tryptophan-rich foods** to promote relaxation and sleep.

Sleepy suppers

Porridge with soya milk, raspberries, flaked almonds and cinnamon

Goat's/sheep's milk yoghurt, toasted oats, chopped Brazil nuts and raspberries

7 Learning to 'switch off'

An overactive mind and inability to '**switch off**' is often blamed for lack of sleep, so it's not surprising that **relaxation strategies** are common interventions for insomnia. Anxiety, stress and depression are among the most common causes of insomnia, so it's understandable that many 'remedies' are based upon relaxation and **meditation** techniques. Research has shown that changing your sleep environment and bedtime behaviour is one of the most effective ways of combating insomnia.

Counting sheep is a form of meditation and visualization, although researchers at the University of Oxford found that visualizing a relaxing scene was more effective

....

In this chapter you will learn about relaxation, meditation and other techniques to help you sleep.

There are various **relaxation techniques** and treatments, most of them requiring 20 minutes or more of practice before going to bed. Within each of these practices, there are several different techniques that may be used:

* meditation
* visualization
* relaxation response
* biofeedback
* progressive muscle relaxation
* hypnosis
* cognitive behavioural therapy.

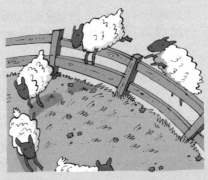

Meditation

The aim of meditation is to 'quieten' the mind. It usually takes several weeks before you have sufficiently mastered the techniques to ease insomnia, but research does appear to support the value of regular meditation for improving sleep, so it's worth persevering with it.

Several studies show that regular meditation results in elevated levels of **melatonin** – the neurotransmitter that stimulates **sleep**. If meditation increases **melatonin** levels – possibly as a result of increased **serotonin** production – then you may be able to induce relaxation and boost **sleep**.

For maximum benefit, try to **meditate** for 20–30 minutes before you go to sleep using a technique that feels comfortable for you.

Visualization

This involves imagining a **relaxing scene** such as a tropical island – the more vivid the image, the more effective it will be, so you should involve as many **senses** as possible, for example imagine looking at the sea, feeling the breeze, listening to the waves, smelling the salty air …

Listening to a **relaxation CD** can help with visualization and help you to 'switch off', relax and sleep. You can listen to examples on the Internet or in a music shop – we all react differently to different sounds, and you need to see what helps you to relax. Popular sounds include:

* ocean waves
* waterfalls
* rain
* birds.

Sounds like this can act as '**white noise**' and mask other noises that may wake you up during the night, so you may wish to keep the CD on at a low volume to help you stay asleep through the night.

Relaxation response

This is a mind/body technique based upon **transcendental meditation**. It is usually practised for 10–20 minutes, three to four times weekly. You might find it useful to do before bedtime each evening:

1 Relax in a comfortable, quiet place and close your eyes.
2 'Belly breathe' slowly, inhaling through the nose and out through the mouth, allowing the stomach to rise and fall with each breath.
3 Choose a peaceful or meaningful word or phrase and repeat it with each exhalation.
4 If your mind wanders, just take a deep breath and start again.
5 At the end of your 'meditation' sit quietly, slowly becoming aware of your surroundings.

78

Biofeedback therapy

This can help to focus the mind on something other than anxiety about not sleeping, simultaneously inducing a type of **meditation** as the mind focuses on **physiological parameters** such as **pulse or breathing rate**.

In **biofeedback therapy**, sensors are connected to a machine and placed on your body to measure various parameters such as heart rate, blood pressure and muscle tension. The machine then produces pictures or sounds to help you control your breathing and body responses, and you can then use these images at bedtime to help reduce your heart rate and/or breathing, which can help you get to sleep.

Progressive muscle relaxation

This technique helps to relax the muscles. Try this in bed to reduce muscle tension and aid relaxation:

* Tense the facial muscles, squeezing the eyes shut, clenching the teeth, grimacing – and hold for 8 seconds.
* Exhale and relax all facial muscles completely.
* Now tense the neck and shoulder muscles, holding for 8 seconds, then relax completely.
* Work down the body … chest, abdomen, arms one at a time, buttocks, legs one at a time, ending with the feet.

With practice, you can shorten this, tensing and relaxing the muscles in four phases:

* face
* neck, shoulders and arms
* abdomen and chest
* buttocks, legs and feet.

Hypnosis and NLP

Hypnosis This aims to suggest solutions and techniques to the **unconscious mind**, once possible causes of insomnia have been explored. The unconscious mind is more open to suggestions: during hypnosis, a suggestion or metaphor may be given to you that reduces tension and sets up the expectation of a good night's sleep.

Neuro-linguistic programming (NLP) Often used in hypnotherapy, NLP aims to flip things around in the unconscious mind; for example, things that may have caused anxiety – and therefore sleeplessness – would instead create relaxation after NLP. This is achieved by linking the thing causing anxiety with a word or image that directs your unconscious mind to calming your thoughts.

Hypnotherapy also uses **visualization**, and may enable you to use **self-hypnosis** and **deep relaxation techniques**, sometimes using a relaxation or hypnosis CD, to help you sleep.

Cognitive behavioural therapy (CBT)

CBT aims to reduce the brain activity associated with anxiety that causes insomnia. If you become anxious about not sleeping, this in itself causes insomnia.

Cognitive techniques help you identify and replace **negative thoughts** about sleep with positive ones. If this reduces anxiety about not sleeping, you may relax more and get to sleep.

For example, 'I won't be able to function tomorrow if I don't sleep soon' is replaced with 'I'm not getting much sleep tonight but I'll still be able to function tomorrow.'

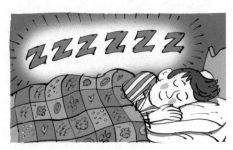

Paradoxical intention

This is CBT that helps retrain fears of not sleeping by doing the opposite of the behaviour that is causing anxiety. For example, if you worry about not being able to sleep long before bedtime, rather than preparing to go to sleep, you deliberately prepare to stay awake.

Another cognitive technique is **sleep restriction** or **sleep scheduling**. This improves '**sleep efficiency**' by reducing the time in bed to the actual amount of sleep you currently get. If you sleep for 5 hours a night but spend 8 hours in bed, you gradually decrease the time spent in bed until you are sleeping for most of it. This aims to increase **sleep drive** and help you enter **deep sleep** more quickly. Once you are sleeping for all the time you spend in bed, the amount of time in bed is gradually increased again each week.

8 Alternative therapies

Many people are seeking **alternative remedies** for health issues these days, and insomnia is a popular example of this. As sleep disturbance is a symptom of something else, and not a condition in its own right, this may be a good step forwards – taking sleeping pills may get you to sleep but it does not deal with the underlying cause of the insomnia.

However, an alternative therapy should also aim to deal with the cause of the insomnia, rather than just the insomnia itself. At least with these therapies, you won't suffer the side effects arising from prescription medications for insomnia.

Chronic insomnia can be a symptom of depression, heart disease or diabetes, so it's important to see your doctor if you are having trouble sleeping

In this chapter, you will learn about the alternative therapies that may be used for insomnia.

Examples of alternative therapies that are regularly used or effective for insomnia include:

* aromatherapy
* homeopathy
* acupuncture and acupressure
* reflexology
* yoga
* herbal medicine
* Chinese medicine
* ayurvedic medicine
* phototherapy or bright light therapy.

Any experience that is relaxing and enjoyable, such as a **massage**, may also enhance relaxation and sleep. Sometimes therapies are undertaken alongside orthodox interventions, in which case they are called complementary therapies.

Aromatherapy

Aromatherapy is the use of essential oils and other aromatic natural botanical oils to promote psychological and physical well-being. Unless inability to relax is the cause of your insomnia, aromatherapy will not cure insomnia or its root cause, but using calming and relaxing essential oils before your bedtime may help you to fall asleep faster and stay asleep.

Aromatherapy oils that may help you to relax and sleep include **chamomile** and **lavender**. Essential oils are very concentrated and can be potent. To ensure safe use:

1 Do not put undiluted essential oils on your skin.
2 Use only small amounts, as essential oils are absorbed through the skin.
3 If you have a medical condition, consult a qualified practitioner before using essential oils, as some oils should not be used by people with certain conditions.

Relaxing essential oils such as chamomile, lavender and lemon balm may heighten the effect of sleeping pills or sedatives

Lavender has been used for centuries to aid sleep. It has been found to increase deep sleep and increase the length of sleep. There are several ways in which you can use lavender to help you sleep:

- ☑ inhaling during visualization
- ☑ inhaling while using the relaxation response
- ☑ using lavender-scented bath products in your pre-bed bath routine
- ☑ adding lavender oil to your bath water
- ☑ dropping lavender essential oil on to a handkerchief to inhale as you lie in bed
- ☑ putting a lavender sachet under or in your pillow
- ☑ adding a few drops in water to a vaporizer and spray into your bedroom
- ☑ drinking a lavender tea infusion before retiring to bed.

Homeopathic remedies

Many individuals benefit from homeopathic remedies, but systematic reviews measuring the effectiveness of homeopathic remedies for insomnia have concluded that further research needs to be done to test their efficacy. After a consultation taking into account an individual's physical, emotional and intellectual make-up, an experienced homeopath may prescribe homeopathic remedies for insomnia.

Such a remedy will aim to allay the cause of the insomnia, thereby having a positive knock-on effect upon your sleep pattern. For example, a well-known anti-anxiety remedy is **nux vomica**: if anxiety was thought to be causing insomnia, this remedy might be prescribed to reduce the anxiety, and therefore the insomnia.

Homeopathic remedies can be bought online or from health stores, although an appointment with a qualified homeopath should provide you with a more useful prescription than an off-the-shelf product.

Acupuncture

Some reports suggest that **acupuncture** may have up to a 90% success rate in reducing insomnia. It involves very fine needles being inserted into the skin at specific acupuncture points – possibly stimulating production of **serotonin** to promote relaxation and sleep.

The results of clinical trials have indicated improvements in **sleep quality** in insomniacs, although additional research is required before its effectiveness can be conclusively proven.

Acupressure may also enhance sleep. An acupressure practitioner stimulates the same pressure points used in acupuncture, but with finger pressure.

One study on acupuncture at Pittsburgh University found that 5 weeks of acupuncture increased the secretion of melatonin in the evening, and thus increased total sleep time

Reflexology

It is not well understood how **reflexology** works, but some reflexologists believe that it may affect the nervous system, reducing insomnia by stimulating or rebalancing the nervous system, resulting in normalizing hormone or neurotransmitter release. Others believe that reflexology breaks down deposits in the feet, which decongests energy pathways and stimulates better energy flow through meridian pathways in the body. Perhaps the **relaxation** and enhanced **sense of well-being** that can come from a reflexology massage simply increases serotonin levels (the 'happy hormone'), reducing anxiety, a key cause of insomnia. If it improves your insomnia, it doesn't really matter how it works!

Exercise

Regular exercise can induce physical – and mental – tiredness and relaxation, helping you to go to sleep and enjoy more deep sleep. Several studies show that exercise can improve sleep. Exercise such as **t'ai chi** and **yoga** include a form of mental '**meditation**'.

Through its focus on the breathing and body positioning, and with its emphasis on breathing control, meditation and stretching the muscles, yoga may provide the perfect exercise antidote to insomnia. A study at Harvard University found that practising yoga daily for 8 weeks improved total sleep time and reduced the time taken to fall asleep.

> **TOP TIP**
> Don't do vigorous exercise within 3 or 4 hours of bedtime as it stimulates the sympathetic nervous system, elevates body temperature and could interfere with sleep.

Phototherapy

Phototherapy or **bright light therapy** optimizes **melatonin secretion** from the pineal gland, helping you to 'reset your body clock' by providing high-intensity light during daytime hours and darkness at night-time.

Circadian rhythm disorders

If you fall asleep early in the evening but wake too early you may have **advanced sleep phase syndrome** – having more light in the evening may help.

If you struggle to fall to sleep but can't rise in the morning you may have **delayed sleep phase syndrome** – try using a **bright light box** between 6 am and 9 am.

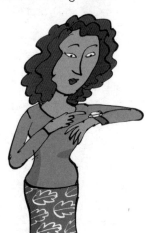

● Set a regular time to go to bed, and a regular time to wake up to reset your body clock

Resetting your body clock

- ☑ Rise at a specific time daily regardless of the previous night's sleep.
- ☑ Submit yourself to bright light at your ideal wake time – this helps you wake in the morning and sleep in the evening.
- ☑ Get plenty of bright light during the day from sunlight or a bright light box.
- ☑ To deepen sleep, restrict sleep to only as much as you need to feel refreshed.
- ☑ If you drop off too early and/or wake too early, get more light in the evening.
- ☑ To elicit sleep at night, ensure dim lighting throughout the evening.

TOP TIP

Don't wear sunglasses if you don't need to – they can block up to 80% of the sunlight entering the eyes and affect your circadian rhythm.

9 Herbs to help

Herbal medicine aims to allay the *underlying cause* of insomnia, rather than simply aid sleep. Herbs have been used for their calming and relaxing properties for centuries, and can be taken as **herbal teas and infusions**, **tinctures** and **capsules**, or added to **baths** or **massage oils**. Many plants have **sedative actions** – those commonly used to aid sleep are valerian, chamomile, hops, lavender, St John's wort, passionflower and lemon balm.

New European legislation means that only herbs assessed by the Medicine and Healthcare Products Regulatory Agency can be sold – look for this logo on approved herbal products.

In this chapter you will learn how you might make use of herbal remedies for insomnia.

Herbal safety

Some herbs **interact with medications** – check with your doctor or a qualified herbalist. Sedative herbs are likely to have **cumulative effects** if taken with drugs for anxiety, depression or insomnia. If you experience any **side effects**, stop taking the herb immediately and notify your doctor or herbalist. Herbs also **interact with each other** (and other supplements) – avoid mixing herbs or consult a qualified practitioner for advice.

Check with your doctor or a qualified medical herbalist if you are **pregnant** or **breastfeeding**.

TOP TIP
Herbs used for insomnia often have a sedative effect so take them before bedtime and not when any level of alertness is required.

Valerian

There are many herbs used to help **insomnia**; each one contains different active constituents with differing properties. For example, for insomnia caused by **stress** or **anxiety**, herbs such as **hops** or **valerian** may be used as these relax the nervous system.

Valerian was used for insomnia in ancient Greece and Rome, and is now used as an over-the-counter insomnia remedy in some European countries. **Anxiety** (a common cause of insomnia) can result from an imbalance in neurotransmitters, and valerian appears to increase the availability of a calming neurotransmitter called **gamma-aminobutyric acid (GABA)** in a similar way to diazepam, which increases GABA activity. Therefore, it should not be taken with sedatives, antihistamines, antidepressants or alcohol. However, unlike many drugs, valerian is not thought to be addictive or cause morning grogginess, although it is not recommended that it be taken for more than 3 months at a time.

Valerian notes

* You can drink valerian tea or take the herb as a supplement or liquid extract.
* Take valerian within an hour of bedtime.
* It may take up to 4 weeks to have any effect.
* Side effects may include indigestion, headache, palpitations and dizziness.
* It may cause excessive daytime drowsiness if taken with medication or other herbs.
* Consultation with a qualified herbalist is recommended.

Chamomile and hops

Chamomile is also commonly used for insomnia, and is considered to be safe, with no known adverse effects. Chamomile is a gentle remedy – a **mild sedative** that may reduce anxiety and relieve muscle tension and spasms. It can be taken as chamomile tea or added to the bath, and can be mixed in equal parts with hops.

Hops have a relaxing and **sleep-inducing** action and may be good for insomnia caused by **restlessness** or **anxiety**. You can drink hops in tea and infusions, or add them to the bath.

Hops, **valerian** and **passionflower** are said to be the three most reliable herbs for insomnia, and they also work well together.

You may benefit from simply having a cup of chamomile tea 1–2 hours before going to bed

St John's wort

Although insomnia can be a side effect of **St John's wort,** it is commonly taken to reduce insomnia and mild depression. It is thought to work through increasing the concentration or effectiveness of **serotonin** in the brain, enhancing a feeling of well-being. This can reduce anxiety, which may result in better relaxation and sleep. Increased serotonin levels may also enhance **melatonin** production, prompting sleep. This may be an effective remedy if you think that your insomnia is related to depression.

You can take St John's wort as a tea, supplement or tincture, but it should not be taken with antidepressants, and it can affect the action of other medications, including the contraceptive pill, so check with your doctor before trying it.

Passionflower

Passionflower can help to calm **anxiety** and relieve **pain** and **muscular spasms**. It may work as valerian does, by increasing GABA levels to enhance relaxation, and/or inhibit serotonin breakdown, reducing anxiety. It may be combined with valerian or lemon balm.

✳ Drink one to two cups of **passionflower tea** or infusion before bedtime.
✳ Take 30–60 drops of passionflower as a **tincture** 45 minutes before bed.
✳ Passionflower is also available as **tablets**.

Cautions

✗ *Passionflower may cause dizziness, nausea, drowsiness, vomiting or irregular muscle action.*
✗ *Don't take it if you are pregnant or breastfeeding.*
✗ *Limit use to 1 month, or as advised by a herbalist.*

Passionflower was used by the Aztecs as a sedative and analgesic

Lemon balm

Lemon balm is considered to be a 'calming' herb, used since the Middle Ages to reduce stress and improve sleep. Few studies have been done on lemon balm and insomnia, but it is often added to insomnia remedies with other herbs.

* Add a quarter to one teaspoonful of dried lemon balm to hot water for lemon balm tea.
* Take as a tincture: 40–90 drops three times daily.
* Add dried lemon balm leaves to bath infusions.
* Take lemon balm capsules.
* Use lemon balm essential oil for an aromatherapy bath or apply topically.

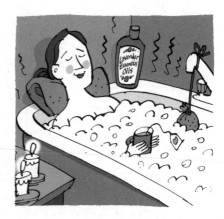

Using herbal remedies

Drinking a **herbal tea** half an hour before bedtime may help you sleep.
Adding a little honey may enhance the taste of some herbal teas. Try any
of these:

* chamomile
* lime blossom (maybe
  with a little skullcap)
* orange blossom
* peppermint leaves
* passionflower
* hops
* valerian
* St John's wort
* fennel seeds
* lavender
* fir needle.

Sleep-inducing remedy
Mix two teaspoons of each herb
(see below) together, then add up
to a tablespoon of the mixture to
a mug of boiling water.

Herb mix: valerian root, lemon
balm, lavender, hops, chamomile.

Making a herbal infusion

1 Add boiling water to herb(s) and leave to brew for 30 minutes.
2 Drink one or two cups 30–60 minutes before bedtime.

You can also add a herbal infusion to a **warm bath** – pour in a litre of strained herbal infusion, or fill a **muslin bag** with herbs, tying it around the tap so that the hot water runs through it. Try **chamomile, lavender** or **valerian**.

Herbal baths

A warm bath can enhance the sedative properties of herbs:

- ☑ Warm water releases the fragrance of the herbs.
- ☑ Heat can activate the properties of some herbs.
- ☑ Heat opens pores, enhancing the action of essential oils and infusions on the skin.

10 Perfect sleep plan

Dealing successfully with insomnia involves:

* figuring out what is causing it
* making changes to your lifestyle or health that enable you to sleep.

Begin with straightforward explanations for your insomnia first, and try to remedy those with equally simple changes, such as reducing or cutting out **caffeine**.

There may be more than one reason for your insomnia – and more than one remedy. You may benefit from keeping a **sleep diary** for a while – this may help you determine what is affecting your sleep, and also help you to measure the success of any changes you make.

This chapter will help you to create a perfect sleep plan from tips throughout this book.

Sleep diary questions

* What were your sleeping times?
* Did you get to sleep easily? How long did it take to get to sleep?
* Did you wake during the night? If so, how many times? Did you get back to sleep easily?
* Do you know what woke you? If you can pinpoint what is waking you, you may be able to do something about it.
* What time did you wake up?
* How refreshed did you feel?

Having a scoring system – maybe 1 to 5 – for getting to sleep, staying asleep and sleep quality can help you to monitor your insomnia and measure the effectiveness of any changes you make

Other things to include in your sleep diary

* How much coffee/tea/chocolate/energy drinks did you consume?
* Did you drink alcohol?
* Did you exercise in the evening?
* Did you nap during the day or evening?
* How stressed or anxious were you feeling?

Answers to these questions in conjunction with your sleep pattern may provide possible reasons for your insomnia. Lifestyle habits such as eating and drinking certain things, exercise times or napping during the day can be changed to see if this will improve your insomnia. If you can't see a link, take your sleep diary to your doctor or health practitioner – they may be able to see a connection.

Prevention is better than cure

Rather than being prepared for when you wake up – for example, with a glass of water at your bedside, see if you can prevent it …

If you wake up **thirsty**, reduce **salt** intake during the day – don't add salt to food or when cooking, and limit your intake of cheese, Marmite, crisps, salted nuts and packaged foods. Reduce your alcohol intake too, as this can also increase thirst.

If you wake up to empty your bladder, drink more fluid early in the day and less later on. Avoid caffeinated drinks and alcohol **(diuretics)**, which stimulate urine production. If this problem persists, you should see your doctor.

If you wake up hungry, try having a supper rich in **slow-release carbohydrates** such as **oats**.

Create the right environment

☑ Keep the bedroom well ventilated.
☑ The bedroom temperature should be cool.
☑ Use restful colours in the bedroom décor.
☑ Keep your bedroom tidy and uncluttered.
☑ Don't work or eat in the bedroom, keep it for sleep and sex.
☑ Use curtains or blackout blinds to shut out light to help you get to sleep, stay asleep and not wake up early.
☑ Cover your clock if you clock watch while trying to sleep.
☑ Have sleep aids in your bedside drawer: eye mask, ear plugs, relaxation CD, book, lavender oil.

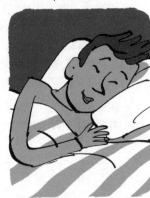

● Create the perfect bedroom environment for sleep …

During the day...

☑ To set your biological clock, get up at the same time daily, regardless of how much sleep you have had, or whether you have to go to work or not.

☑ Figure out how much sleep you need to feel fully revitalized and plan bedtime and wake time around this.

☑ Reduce your caffeine and alcohol intake.

☑ Don't sleep during the day.

☑ Get plenty of exposure to light during the day.

☑ Exercise daily but not too late in the evening.

TOP TIP

If you're happy to go with your natural circadian rhythm ...

'Night owls' go to bed later and rise later.

'Early larks' retire earlier and rise earlier.

This may reduce anxiety about your sleep pattern.

Sweet dreams bedtime routine

- ☑ Keep the lights dimmed through the evening time.
- ☑ Avoid eating big meals or spicy foods.
- ☑ Don't smoke before bedtime.
- ☑ Avoid alcohol.
- ☑ Relax with gentle yoga, a warm bath, a little reading …
- ☑ Have a milky drink or herbal tea before bedtime.
- ☑ Use a herb pillow or essential bath oils.
- ☑ Go to bed at the same time each night.
- ☑ Write a to-do list for tomorrow to clear your mind.
- ☑ Only go to bed if you are tired.
- ☑ Close the doors and windows to shut out noise.
- ☑ Close the blackout blinds to achieve complete darkness.
- ☑ Wear ear plugs or an eye mask if required.

Music

Listening to **music** or an **audiobook** combines a number of psychological tools in a simple activity. Listening to **music** can have the following effects:

* It can aid visualization.
* Some types of music may aid meditation.
* Some types of classical music act as 'white noise', enabling the mind to switch off and relax.
* Music can reduce anxiety and aid relaxation.

Music has been found to improve sleep quality, decrease nightly wakenings, lengthen sleep time and increase sleep quality.

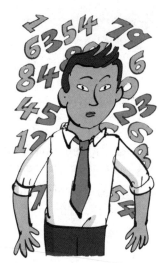

● A busy mind is not conducive to dropping off to sleep ... listen to relaxing music or an audiobook before going to sleep

Audiobooks

Audiobooks may enable you to transport yourself into another place and time, with the benefits of …

* taking your mind off any worries you may have (reducing anxiety)
* visualizing what's happening in the book (visualization)
* stopping you from clock watching (reducing stress about not getting to sleep)
* creating a meditative state of mind as some voice tones can act as 'white noise' and help put you to sleep (meditation).

Headphones may be uncomfortable if you're lying in bed (and falling asleep wearing them), so invest in a CD player instead, unless you'll be keeping someone else awake.

If you still can't get to sleep ...

* If it takes longer than 20–30 minutes to get to sleep, **get up** and go to another room and read or do something else, and try again later.
* **Don't watch the clock** as this will only make you anxious.
* If something is on your mind, **write a list of worries/things to do**, then forget about it until morning.
* **Inhale** a relaxing fragrance from a herb pillow, homeopathic remedy or aromatherapy oil.
* Use a ceiling fan or relaxation CD as 'white noise' to switch off your mind.
* Try **meditation, visualization, progressive muscle relaxation** or any cognitive behavioural techniques you have practised.

Further reading

* www.altmedrev.com/publications/12/2/101.pdf (research article on restless legs syndrome)
* www.britishsnoring.co.uk – for information on sleep apnoea and snoring to help snorers and their sleeping partners
* www.emedicinehealth.com/insomnia/article_em.htm
* www.helpguide.org/life/sleep_apnea.htm
* www.helpguide.org/life/sleep_aids_medication_insomnia_treatment.htm
* www.moodjuice.scot.nhs.uk/sleepproblems.asp
* www.nhs.co.uk/Conditions/Insomnia/Pages/Introduction.aspx
* www.sleepcouncil.com – promotes the benefits of sleeping well and provides information leaflets on sleep and beds
* www.sleeppcouncil.org.uk
* www.sleepfoundation.org – an American website with information on sleep and sleep disorders